The Skinny Book

The 6-Step Methodology for Weight Management

Ayaz Virji, MD

Verona Publishing, Inc.
P.O. Box 24071
Edina, Minnesota 55424

www.veronapublishing.com

Verona Publishing is pleased to present The Skinny Book, if you are interested in purchasing more copies or if you are interested in books on other topics.

Books can be ordered at www.veronapublishing.com

When ordering in bulk email us the type and number of books required at info@veronapublishing.com

Coming soon to Verona Publishing

Putting the Pieces Together, a book dealing with Borderline Personality Disorder.

And in the fiction category a moving story by author Nancy DeRosa, *There's No Place like home*.

Watch for these titles and many more at www.veronapublishing.com or wherever books are sold.

For questions or comments, contact us at info@veronapublishing.com

Cover photo by David Ewart Photography

Design and layout by Janie Nordberg

The Skinny Book 2004

Published by Verona Publishing, Inc., P.O. Box 24071, Edina, Minnesota 55424

Library of Congress Cataloging-in-Publication Data:

Library of Congress Control Number: 2004106948

ISBN 0-9667037-7-4

Verona Publishing, Inc.
P.O. Box 24071
Edina, Minnesota 55424

www.veronapublishing.com

For my wife,

Without her loving support and dedication I would never have

Been able to complete this work.

For my kids,

Thank you for teaching me how to modify my behavior

so I could report it to others.

For my patients,

It is truly an honor for me to be involved in your medical care.

I will always do my best to serve you

With the quality care, dignity, and respect you deserve.

Disclosure

The author has no commercial affiliations or associations to disclose. At the time of Publication, Dr. Virji did not receive any financial support from any individual, group, or company. The commercial products mentioned in the book can be substituted for any like branded item. Specific names or brands were used out of convention and illustration only.

Acknowledgments

First and foremost, I would like to thank God for giving me the capacity to serve others. My life will only be successful if I am bringing good to those around me. I would like to thank my parents for all they have done for me to bring me where I am today. Thanks to my family and friends who read and helped me revise the many rough drafts of this book. Thanks to my loving wife whose support was enduring and always there in times of greatest need.

I would also like to thank Morton Plant Mease Primary Care. I am proud to be part of such a quality and committed organization whose focus has always been and always will be on the patient first. Since I first interviewed with the organization, I was impressed with its ethical and professional approach to patient care, and I look forward to the many years ahead as a practicing Morton Plant Mease physician.

I thank Verona Publishing for giving me the opportunity to create this work and distribute it to those it can best serve. Thanks Monty. We live in a great country and have overcome many large hurdles throughout our history as Americans. The obesity epidemic does threaten us; however, we will address it thoroughly, intelligently, and confidently and overcome it in the end as well. This book will help us toward that end.

About the Author

Ayaz Virji, MD is a family physician at Morton Plant Mease Primary Care in Clearwater, FL. He received his MD from Georgetown University Medical School and completed his residency training in family medicine at Duke University Medical Center. He has a special interest in obesity medicine and runs a very successful weight management program in his current clinical practice. He is a registered provider with The American Obesity Association and is committed to fighting the obesity epidemic in the country head-on. He is a member of the American Medical Association, The American Academy of Family Physicians, The North American Association for the Study of Obesity, and The American Society of Bariatric Physicians.

Table of Contents

Part I

Obesity as an Epidemic

As Americans, when we speak of medical diseases the first thing that comes to our minds are heart disease, strokes, and cancer. And why not, these diseases are the leading causes of death and suffering nationwide, and perhaps worldwide. We all have friends or family members who are suffering from or were lost to a heart attack or a various type of cancer. We never hear of those people who are suffering from or who died of obesity. That would be absurd, right?

Wrong. Obesity is one of the leading causes of death and suffering in this country (1,2). Obesity is a major risk factor for heart disease, stroke, diabetes, colon cancer, breast cancer, ulcer diseases, gallbladder disease, osteoarthritis, major depressive disorders, and chronic pain disorders to name a few. Obese patients suffer from more chronic medical conditions than patients of normal weight and body mass index. Obese patients are harder to perform major surgeries on due to anatomical barriers. The list goes on and on.

Given the above facts and the fact that over 60% of American adults are either obese or overweight, I think the point is clearly made that obesity is an epidemic in this country leading to significant medical complications and even death (3). It acts as a thread that binds together many medical diseases of different sorts that overwhelmingly attacks an individual who suffers from it. Therefore, weight management issues are of crucial importance to both medical and non-medical personnel across the board. Its importance permeates even to the national level.

I hope I have convinced you that obesity as a disease is at the same level of importance as heart disease, diabetes, and even breast cancer. In fact, it is an independent risk factor for all three of these. Dealing with weight management is like repairing a shipping vessel before sending it out to sea. Treating a heart attack or stroke is like rescuing the passengers from the sinking ship. Why not focus on fixing the leaks first and preventing the catastrophe before it happens? This, of course is a simple analogy. Heart disease and strokes are multi-factorial medical diseases with many different risk factors involved. Nevertheless, the point remains true that by "repairing" obesity, the prevalence of heart disease, strokes, diabetes, and cancer are guaranteed to significantly decline in this country.

As a physician, I deal with obesity and weight management on a daily basis. My methods have been extremely successful in helping a significant proportion of my patients "repair" their obesity. Unfortunately, in the medical field, weight management does not get attributed the amount of importance and time it really deserves.

As an example of this dilemma, in primary care we deal with upper respiratory infections, heart disease, diabetes, fractures, rashes, newborn exams, liver disease, asthma, migraine headaches, etc. In a typical day, your average family physician will deal with all of the above plus about 20-30 more medical issues for patients. On top of that is the endless amount of paperwork, charting, and coding required by insurance companies and the legal system that has to be dealt with. It can be quite overwhelming.

You can imagine your average physician's response when a patient inquires about weight loss. "Diet and exercise" is the answer. But what exactly does that mean? What diet is best for you? How will you get there? What else is required? How will weight be maintained? What type of medical surveillance or technology can help?

These are all issues that need to be thoroughly addressed before weight loss can be achieved and maintained successfully. Your physician will be so busy dealing with many different, more immediate problems, as well as fulfilling mandatory documenting, coding, and administrative paperwork, it's no wonder why he has little enthusiasm when at the end of you visit you mention to him, "And doctor, about my weight...?"

Obesity is a multi-factorial disease, as are most diseases we encounter in medicine. Weight management requires a significant amount of time and energy from both sides. As a patient, you wouldn't end a visit with you doctor by saying, "Oh, and about my chest pain." Obesity, like chest pain, merits the complete attention of your doctor and should be the sole focus of your visit when addressing it.

Part II

The Purpose of this Book

The purpose of this book is to introduce you to my 6-step methodology for weight loss and more importantly weight maintenance. I collectively refer to these two very distinct features under the banner of "weight management." My methods have been extremely successful for my patients.

This is not a diet book. There are a number of good diets already out there. There is no point in reinventing the wheel. I'll teach you more about these under the chapter of "Diet Selection." In order to be successful you must read this book from cover to cover and understand what is being taught.

I will take you through the physiology of weight reduction and weight maintenance. You will learn about the many co-morbidities of obesity and important medically related topics. We will use principles of biochemistry as well as psychology to help you achieve your goal. Patients in my clinic have a near 100% success rate for weight loss and weight maintenance. I will do my best to help teach you all you need to know to share the same level of success through one simple book.

The best part about this book is that you're going to learn all you need to know in record time! I have purposely made this book as short as possible for quick reading and easy referencing. You don't need a 500 page book to describe to you how to lose weight. In the words of Albert Einstein, "Things should be made as simple as possible, but not simpler."

Now, let us begin our journey with the most important concept of them all. Obesity is a multi-factorial disease.

Part III

Why My Methods Work: The Multi-factorial Approach

In the Medical field, the majority of diseases we treat have multi-factorial etiologies. What this means is that there is no one thing causing them. Instead, many different things are involved to cause you to develop a certain disease. Consider the following examples.

Heart disease is not caused by increased cholesterol alone. Other modifiable risk factors besides high cholesterol that lead to it include: OBESITY, high blood pressure, sedentary lifestyle, diabetes, and elevated homocysteine levels (family history, age, and gender are not modifiable risk factors). Factors that lead to colon cancer include: OBESITY, high-fat, low-fiber diet, chronic constipation, and family history. Factors involved in gallstone formation include: OBESITY, age, fertility status, and gender. The list goes on and on. We could fill an entire book just listing all the specific risk factors for the different diseases out there. The point being, no one particular thing has total say over whether or not you develop or can control a certain disease. There are many forces at play, and successful disease control involves recognition and treatment of the many different variables involved.

Obesity is no different. Risk factors include: a sedentary lifestyle, poor diet, certain medical conditions (hypothyroidism, anemia, certain medications), and depression. I would also extend this list to include unhealthy congnitive barriers and detrimental behavior patterns. My 6-Step Methodology deals with every modifiable aspect of obesity not just diet and exercise alone, which is why it is so successful. Here is a summary of how we do it:

1) **Medical Screening**: The first step is to ensure that there is no underlying disease process involved that is sabotaging your weight loss efforts. You will need your doctor's help with this.

2) **Patient Education**: Knowledge is power. Once you see how the pieces of the puzzle fit, your goal of weight management becomes much easier to obtain.

3) **Diet Selection/Exercise Review**: Choosing between the traditional quantitative balanced diet versus the new modified-carbohydrate diets can be quite confusing. I'll help you out with this.

4) **Cognitive Principles**: Certain misconceptions about weight loss create significant barriers to weight management. We will eradicate these and prevent them from returning.

5) **Behavioral Issues**: We'll discuss some behavioral patterns specific to healthy weight management.

6) **Weight Maintenance**: Includes intensive follow-ups, surveillance of medical diseases, and surveillance of weight loss.

Now, let's begin the 6-Step Methodology for Weight Management. Success is awaiting you at the turn of a page!

Part IV

Step 1: Medical Screening

I have already shown you that obesity is related to many diseases and by preventing it you will add many quality years to your life. Before you begin the process of weight management, you have to be certain that you don't have any medical conditions that are going to slow down your weight loss. Going to your physician and getting a Complete Physical Exam (your doctor may refer to this as a CPE) is the first step. That should include a head-to-toe exam, appropriate preventive screening, and lab work. The lab work will include a complete blood count (CBC), fasting lipid profile (which is the technical term for a complete cholesterol panel), thyroid level, fasting blood sugar, kidney function tests, and liver function tests (LFT's). Tell your physician that you are beginning a new weight management program and you want to be sure you are healthy enough to do so. Annual physical exams are very informative to both patients and physicians, and I would recommend them to everyone, whether you are trying to lose weight or not.

Hypothyroidism (or low thyroid hormone level) will slow your body's metabolism down. Symptoms of it include obesity, constipation, fatigue, dry skin, and hair loss. Your doctor will order a TSH level (thyroid stimulating hormone) which gives a very precise measure of your thyroid gland's function. A complete blood count (CBC) looks at your blood for any anemia or infections. It also gives insight on certain vitamin and mineral deficiencies by looking at the size, shape, and color of the red blood cells, which can vary with different nutritional deficiencies.

Obesity is the most common cause of a certain liver disease called NASH (non-alcoholic steatohepatitis). This is where fat cells accumulate along the liver leading to inflammation. This can be a risk factor for significant liver disease later in life. By measuring your liver function tests (LFT's) your doctor can check for this. NASH always improves once weight gets down. If you have NASH, once you lose the weight your doctor can reorder the test for you and you will see the improvement for yourself.

Checking your kidney function tests is also very important to get a baseline measure of the various minerals and salts in your blood as well as screen for any kidney disease. Certain diets will make the kidneys work a little harder for a short period of time so you want to make sure they are ready to handle the task. In most otherwise healthy people this is not a problem. In people with compromised kidney function this needs to be watched closely.

Checking your cholesterol is very important as well. According to the National Cholesterol Education Program (NCEP) guidelines all people above the age of twenty should be screened for high cholesterol. If you are overweight it is very likely that your cholesterol is also too high. You need to know what yours is.

Specifically, you need to know what your levels of LDL (bad cholesterol) and HDL (good cholesterol) are. For your LDL, the lower the better; For your HDL, the higher the better. No matter where your cholesterol is now, it's guaranteed to improve once the weight comes off. If you are on a cholesterol lowering medication, you might even be able to come off it once your obesity is repaired. Your doctor can explain to you what your specific cholesterol goals are since it varies from person to person.

If you have any depressive disorder or other psychological disorder you need to discuss that with your doctor and get treatment first. Depressive disorders like Major Clinical Depression can cause what we call psychomotor retardation which basically makes you and your body move with a general slowing and lack of energy. This will slow your metabolism and your weight loss, not to mention be bad for your overall health in general. There are some great medical treatments out there for depression that will make you feel better and also add years to your life. A very important medical study called the SADHEART Trial showed that in patients who suffered a heart attack who had their depression treated lived much longer and were less likely to suffer another heart attack than those who had untreated depression.

Actually, effectively managing your weight with the 6-Step Methodology will have a very positive effect on your mood and energy level overall (4). You'll find that as you lose weight your depression will get better as well. Nevertheless, we do not want any psychological issues hindering our weight management program.

Traditional approaches to weight loss do not even consider these very important medical and psychological factors to weight loss. All patients in my weight management clinic get a complete physical exam (CPE), appropriate lab work, and general medical screening to prepare them for the upcoming weight loss and maintenance. This is one of the reasons why my program is so successful. You need to know how your weight is affecting your own health. We need to be sure there is nothing predisposing you to failure on a biological or psychological level.

I had a patient who came to see me for some help in weight loss who said he had tried everything and had known nothing but failure his entire life. I enrolled him in my program. I checked his thyroid level which happened to be low, and I corrected it. We went through the 6-Step Methodology together, and he successfully lost over 30 lbs. He is down to his ideal body weight and has kept it off. He is currently in step 6 (Weight Maintenance) which is lifelong and prevents you from gaining weight back.

I had another obese patient come to me insisting that her thyroid be checked because she was overweight and claimed she was doing everything right but not losing the weight. She already had her thyroid checked earlier in the year, and it was normal. When I reviewed this with her she began to cry. I immediately noted her cognitive barrier to weight loss. I gave her cognitive and behavioral therapy, enrolled her in my program, and she lost 20 lbs and has thus far kept it off. She is also in step 6 and is feeling happier and healthier than ever before.

Medical screening and surveillance are important parts of the weight management package. Now that you understand their significance, you see why many weight loss programs fail in either losing the weight or keeping the weight off. Even certain medications can hinder weight loss. You need your doctor's help in identifying these barriers so you can cross them and move on. Now, let's move on to Step 2.

Part IV

Step 2: Patient Education

Alright, hold on to your hats! Knowledge is power, and with this chapter I'm going to teach you some of the most important principles and physiologic mechanisms involved in your weight management. When you understand these principles, you will know what your body is doing and why things work the way they do, including why most people gain the weight back after a short, vigorous weight loss program. I usually go over this information with my patients during their first weight management consult. It's amazing how responsive they are to this information. I believe that knowledge of these key principles helps define for people weight loss goals as well as gives the necessary insight of how to correctly lose weight by understanding some fundamental human physiology. We will review the following key concepts:

1) What is a Body Mass Index (BMI)

2) How a low-carb/modified-carb diet really works

3) The Leptin Theory of weight maintenance

Body Mass Index (BMI)

Let's start with the Body Mass Index, otherwise known as the BMI. The BMI is how we define obesity. For adults, it is equal to your weight in kilograms divided by your height in meters squared:

$$\text{BMI} = \frac{\text{Weight (kilograms)}}{\text{Height (meters) squared}}$$

To calculate your weight in kilograms you should check your weight in pounds and then divide that number by 2.2. That will give you your weight in kilograms. Measure your height in centimeters (one inch is equal to 2.54 centimeters) and then divide that number by 100 to get your height in meters. Then, multiply that number by itself to get the height in meters squared. For example:

What is the BMI of a 220 pound person who is 160 cm tall?

220 pounds/2.2 = 100 kg

160 cm/100 = 1.6 meters

1.6 x 1.6 = 2.56 meters squared

BMI = 100/2.56 = 39

Now, here is how you classify your weight based on your BMI:

BMI	Classification
20-25	Normal
25-30	Overweight
30-40	Obese (high risk for many diseases)
> 40	Morbidly Obese (severely high risk)

Our theoretical patient has a BMI of 39 so he fits under the "obese" classification. He is a perfect candidate for the 6-Step Methodology for Weight Management. Why don't you try and calculate your own BMI? Mine is 21.*

The Body Mass Index equation is well-accepted in the medical community as a means of classifying obesity for most adults. It should be noted however, that it is inaccurate for certain populations including pregnant women, children, and body builders. If you fit in one of these categories, you will need to consult your doctor regarding your weight classification.

The low-car/modified-carb diet

Now you know your weight classification. Let's talk a little about the "low-carb phenomenon." From a physiologic standpoint, the low-car/modified-carb diet makes a lot of sense and actually works wonderfully for many people. Of the different low-carb/modified-carb diets my personal favorite is the South Beach Diet (which is actually a modified-carb not low-carb diet). I put about 70% of my patients on this diet. We'll go into the details of why in the next chapter. Here is how the low-carb/modified-carb diet works.

1) Insulin is a hormone secreted by your pancreas, which is basically a gland sitting in the middle of your back behind your stomach. Insulin is responsible for sugar utilization and the converting of extra calories into fat molecules. When insulin levels are high, that causes you to gain weight.

2) Insulin is secreted in response to the intake of sugars. Sugars and carbohydrates are the same thing. They are synonyms (refer to figure 1).

Figure 1

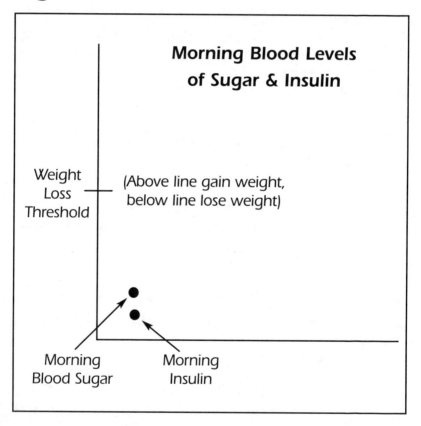

3) When sugar levels, which are the same thing as carbohydrate levels, go up (like after eating that morning muffin or bagel) your pancreas responds by shooting out insulin to get moving on the metabolism of that sugar and the production of fat molecules to store it (figures 2 and 3).

Figure 2

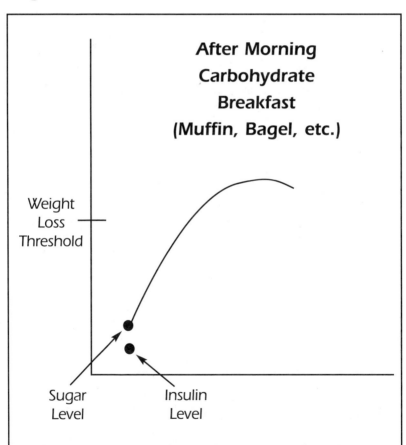

4) As a result, the now high insulin levels cause your body to get hypoglycemic (low-sugar). The rapid rise in insulin has caused the sugar to be moved from the blood into different cells, including fat cells for fat production, so your blood sugar level is now low again (figure 3).

Figure 3

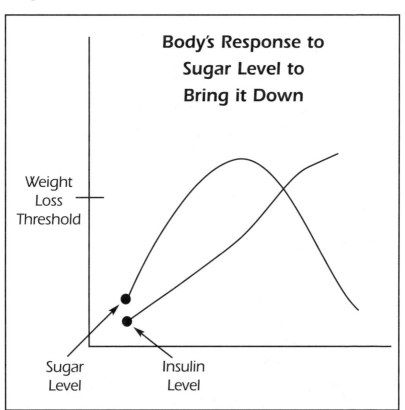

5) Your hypothalamus (which is the part of the brain responsible for appetite control) now senses the low blood sugar and tells your body that you are hungry again.

6) You are now hungry again and eat more either to gain weight or stay the same. This is a vicious cycle that happens throughout the day (figure 4). Remember how you are always hungry one to two hours after eating Chinese food, which is very rich in carbohydrates like noodles, rice, sweet sauces, etc. Well this is what's going on.

Figure 4

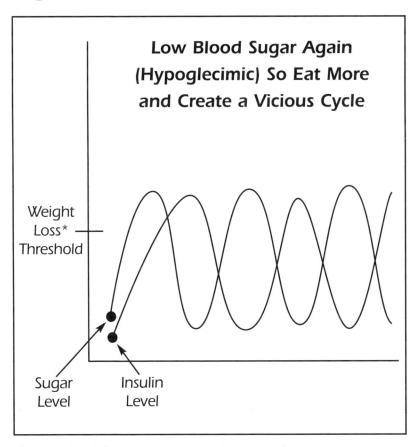

* Note, you never stay below the Weight Loss Threshold, so you never lose weight.

Now, consider the low-carb/modified-carb diet (figure 5). Notice how the lines stay well below the weight threshold line. So your body has no choice but to melt the fat away and lose the weight.

Figure 5

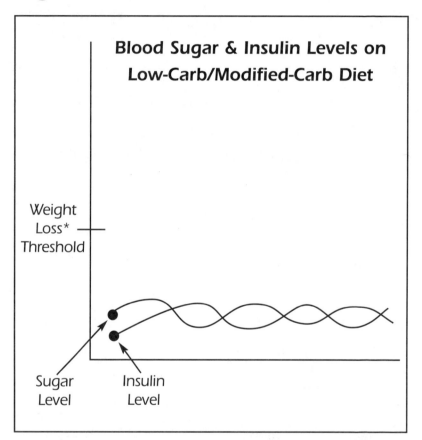

* Note, now you always stay below the Weight Loss Threshold for Sugar and Insulin Levels. Your body has no choice but to melt the pounds away.

Low-carb/modified-carb diets are not for everyone. There are certain medical conditions that may get worse if you have them on a low-carb diet (we'll get into these later). But if you qualify, and most people do, it is a very effective weight loss tool as you can see. You will however need the rest of the steps in this book to effectively "weight manage." I have a number of patients who rebound to prior weight after a short low-carb binge. I implemented the 6-step Methodology and reduced their weight to healthy levels and kept it off.

The Leptin Theory

Now we will discuss the Leptin theory of obesity. This is crucial to understanding not so much the weight loss component of my program, but the maintenance of weight lost, which is of course the most important step of any weight loss program.

Your fat cells secrete a neurohormone called leptin, which acts in the hypothalamus (the part of the brain responsible for appetite control among other things). Leptin acts to inhibit your appetite so you don't feel hungry (5,6). Now, as you lose weight and all your fat cells begin to shrink, your body's leptin concentration goes down because you have less fat cell mass to produce the hormone. Your fat cells are smaller so they secrete less leptin.

Your hypothalamus is not used to the smaller supply of leptin so it tells your body you are hungry. You then eat and gain weight again until your fat cells reach the same size they were before and secrete the same amount of leptin that your hypothalamus is used to seeing. This is why people who lose weight, particularly those who lose it so fast, so often go right back to their previous weight in a matter of weeks to months. You body has this internal signaling pattern, which utilizes leptin concentration as the signal to your brain, to keep your body at a certain pre-set weight. If you fluctuate up or down for a certain time period, your body begins the signaling pattern to correct the fluctuation and return your fat cells back to their previous size, usually resulting in "maintenance of obesity."

Here is how I deal with this little hang-up in the 6-Step Methodology for my patients. First, we choose the diet. Then we lose 10% of your body weight in about 12 weeks. It has been clinically proven that obese patients who lose as little as 10% of their weight have a significant reduction in the risk of developing many serious medical illnesses including coronary heart disease and diabetes (7,8). Even if you do not reach your ideal body weight, BMI between 20 to 25, by losing 10% of weight you get a significant health benefit.

Once that first goal of 10% of weight loss is achieved we reset our goals to a cruise control mode. All efforts at "weight loss" are ceased and diverted exclusively to "weight maintenance." This is a crucial part of the process and is how we deal with the influence of leptin. We stay in this phase for about 12 weeks. During this time, your hypothalamus is now getting used to the lower concentration of leptin. It now resets its receptors for the leptin hormone to the new lower levels and now accepts it as normal and stops that initial powerful force to try and bring you back to your old weight. This is a theoretical model that I feel has much validity and must be dealt with for any weight management program to be successful. After that

12 week weight maintenance phase, we go back to weight loss again if needed. Slow and steady wins the race. Weight management is no different.

You now understand some fundamental principles of weight classification and weight management on the scientific level. This understanding is crucial to your success. Sometimes the medical language can be burdensome. I've tried my best to simplify the explanations the best I could. If you did not understand some parts of the previous discussion please go back and reread those parts. This book is quite short so it shouldn't take you long to do so.

Knowledge is power, and now you are empowered to move on to step 3! Let's choose a diet for you.

Part IV

Step 3: Diet Selection/Exercise

As I mentioned before, this is not a diet book. There are a number of good diets out there, and I do not plan on reinventing the wheel. Let's talk about something more important, diet selection.

There exist only two kinds of diets out there: quantitative diets and qualitative diets. All advertised diets can fit under one of these two categories, or a combination thereof. They are defined below:

1) **Quantitative diet**: a diet that involves the counting of calories. There is no elimination of any one food group. Instead, all food groups are usually consumed in a balanced manner, but the total number of calories consumed are monitored very closely and reduced to obtain weight loss. This is the traditional low-calorie, balanced diet you've probably tried many times in the past.

2) **Qualitative diet**: does not involve the counting of calories. Instead, it involves food group restriction or elimination as in the example of low-carbohydrate or modified-carbohydrate diets. Calories are irrelevant and are not monitored.

With my patients, I discuss the differences between the two types of diets, and we select one together. No two people are created the same. Every person has there own particular biases, eating habits, cravings, lifestyle, medical screening results (which can affect diet selection), and methods that have failed them in the past. We go into this in depth and select the appropriate diet together.

I have to admit that in my clinic I have a very strong tendency to recommend the qualitative diet approach. There exist a number of studies done at a number of reputable institutions that have demonstrated the safety and success of modified carbohydrate dieting (9,10). The diet I generally recommend is The South Beach Diet (the other modified-carb diets out there like The Sugar Busters Diet are probably just as good). I use this diet on about 70% of my patients and have great success with it. It is a modified-carbohydrate diet that focuses on consumption of the good fats and proteins as well as the good carbohydrates, those with the lowest glycemic indexes.

The South Beach Diet utilizes the concept of the glycemic index of foods as the cornerstone of meal planning and selection. The glycemic index of a particular carbohydrate-containing food is basically a measure of the amount of insulin stimulation in the body that results from consumption of that particular food. Since we know that elevated insulin levels lead to appetite stimulation and fat production, foods with the lowest glycemic index are the most desirable. Foods such as rice, potatoes, white bread, and desserts have a very high glycemic index and are avoided in The South Beach Diet. Foods such as cabbage, celery, broccoli, lettuce, and mushrooms have a low glycemic index and can be consumed freely in the diet. In addition, the diet is filled with high quality protein and high quality fats such as those found in chicken, fish, eggs, low-fat cheese, and nuts. The diet is organized into three separate phases, each with its unique list of allowable foods. As you progress through each phase, the food choices become less restrictive. Overall, it's a scientifically sound and very effective way to diet.

Remember figure 5 from the previous chapter and how your insulin levels play a key role in your body's fat content. Well, following The South Beach Diet (or another modified-carb diet like it) will keep your insulin at a low, healthy level that will melt the fat away. In addition, you will avoid low blood sugar levels and by doing so keep your hypothalamus (the appetite control center of the brain) in check, which will work to reduce your appetite and caloric consumption in general. Please refer back to figures 1-5 in the previous chapter if you forgot how this works.

The Atkin's Diet is a similar type of qualitative diet. However, it is a low-carb diet versus The South Beach Diet which is a modified-carb diet. The carbohydrate factor is much more restricted, and the type of fat consumption encouraged, in my opinion, is too heavy in the bad fats (saturated fats), unlike The South Beach Diet which is heavy on the good fats (mono and polyunsaturated fats). Saturated fat turns into LDL (bad cholesterol) in your body and deposits on your various blood vessels to clog your arteries. Mono and polyunsaturated fats (the good fats) increase your level of HDL (good cholesterol) which goes to your arteries and helps strip the cholesterol away, kind of like a roto-rooter cleaning pipes. Although there are a number of success stories with this diet, many physicians have a hard time recommending the diet to their patients because of the heavy saturated fat consumption.

There are certain medical conditions which may preclude you from being on a modified/low-carb diet, which will for the most part be high in protein and fat. So, you'll need to discuss this with your doctor. Some medical conditions that could be potentially worsened by such a diet include chronic renal failure (kidney disease), congestive heart failure (if on diuretic therapy), and peptic ulcer disease. If you have any of these conditions or are pregnant or nursing, you'll need your doctor's guidance on this.

Now, if you are someone who absolutely cannot give up your carbs or has a medical reason not to be on a low-carb/modified-carb diet then the quantitative diet approach may be the one for you. Let me show you how to do this one.

The first step is to calculate the number of calories you can consume a day to get to your goal weight. To do this we need to first calculate your ideal body weight. This formula is essentially the reverse of the BMI (body mass index) formula and is equal to 23 multiplied by your height in meters squared:

Ideal body weight = 23 X (height in meters squared)

This will give you your ideal body weight in kilograms. Multiply this number by 2.2 to get it in pounds. To get your daily caloric allowance you take your ideal body weight in pounds and multiply it by ten:

Caloric allowance = Ideal body weight in pounds X 10

Pretty simple right! Let's practice.

Let's take a person who is 5 ft 10 inches tall and go over our calculations.

5 ft 10 inches = 70 inches

70 inches X 0.0254 meters/inch = 1.74 meters

Our equation for ideal body weight:

Ideal Body Weight = 23 X (height in meters squared)

= 23 X (1.74 squared)

= 69 kilograms

To convert kilograms to pounds, multiply number by 2.2:

69 kilograms X 2.2 = 151 pounds

Caloric allowance = weight in pounds x 10

= 151 pounds X 10

1,510 calories allowed/day

So our 5 ft 10 inch person will need to restrict his daily calorie intake to 1,510 calories/day. This will lead to an average 1-2 pound weight loss per week until he reaches his ideal body weight. Why don't you try calculating your own ideal body weight and daily caloric allowance. Remember, if you're on The South Beach Diet there's no need to count calories. These equations will be irrelevant to you and you can retire your calculators.

Once you've calculated your daily caloric allowance, the second important step in a quantitative diet is to utilize some form of portion controlled meal replacements (PCMR). PCMR are pre-packaged, nutritionally fortified meals or snacks that basically add structure to your diet by doing the calorie counting for you. Popular brands of PCMR include *Slim fast, Glucerna, Lean Cuisine,* and *Healthy Choice.* They are very practical and easy to use particularly when you're on the go (like most of us are) and can easily be substituted for fast food. They are found in most grocery stores nationwide.

Studies show that we underestimate our calorie intake by at least 30% when we are dieting (11). In addition, a number of studies show that people on calorie counting diets who use some form of PCMR lose more weight and, more importantly, keep it off compared to those who don't use them (12,13). Refer to Table 1-3 for sample menus.

Let's talk a moment about dietary fiber. This is particularly important if you are on a quantitative diet. I generally look at fiber as "The Lost Nutrient." In the midst of the grueling war between low-fat diets versus low-carb/mod-carb diets, we have forgotten about the importance of high-fiber foods in the battle against obesity.

Dietary fiber is a form of complex carbohydrate that breaks down very slowly and absorbs a lot of water as it transits through the digestive system. By doing this, it helps prevent insulin surges as well as promotes a sense of fullness and appetite suppression. By the way, it will also keep you regular and help prevent against colon cancer too. Foods high in fiber will help you lose weight, and you'll need to get into the habit of choosing them over their starchy counterparts, even if the calorie counts are the same.

Let's take an example. White bread and wheat bread may have the same amount of calories per slice. However, your body treats them both in very different ways. You will get a blood sugar and insulin spike with the white bread which will leave you hungry one hour later. The high-fiber wheat bread will break down slowly keeping your insulin levels low and keeping you full for longer. The same goes for whole wheat pasta vs regular pasta, wild rice vs white rice, and so on. If you are on a quantitative diet, you need to shop high-fiber and low-calorie, not just low-calorie.

Table 1 (Calorie Counting Diet Menu)

	Calories
Breakfast:	
2 tablespoons Benefiber in 12 oz glass of sugar free ice tea	
Slim Fast Chocolate Royal milkshake	260
Mid-morning Snack:	
Medium sized pear	120
Lunch:	
Lean Cuisine 5-cheeze lasagna	
Diet soft drink	
Sugar free jell-o	350
Mid-afternoon Snack:	
Hershey's 1 gram Sugar Carb bar*	120
Dinner:	
2 tablespoons *Benefiber* in 12 oz glass of water	
Well-balanced reasonable sized meal of your choice	600
Dessert: Low-fat frozen fudge bar	
(or *Slim Fast* Snack Options chocolate bar)	120
Total Calories:	1570

* Hershey's 1 gram Sugar Carb Bar is a great snack for either low/mod-carb diets or quantitative calorie counting diets. It's filled with a whopping 7 grams of fiber and low in calories, not to mention delicious. So enjoy!

Table 2 (Calorie Counting Diet Menu)

	Calories
Breakfast: 2 tablespoons *Benefiber* in 12oz glass of water *Dr. Phil* /shape Up Chocolate Peanut Butter Bar*	250
Mid-morning Snack: Low-fat yogurt and fruit cup	90
Lunch: *Healthy Choice* Chicken Enchilada Diet soft drink Sugar-free jell-o	300
Mid-afternoon Snack: *Hershey's* 1 gram Sugar Carb Bar	120
Dinner: 2 tablespoons *Benefiber* in 12oz glass of *Crystal Light* ice tea Well-balanced reasonable sized meal of your choice	600
Dessert: Low-fat frozen fudge bar	120
Total Calories:	1480

* *I've looked at the various meal replacement breakfast bars on the market and like Dr. Phil's brand the best. It has 6 grams of fiber per bar and tastes great.*

Table 3 (Calorie Counting Diet Menu)

	Calories
Breakfast:	
2 tablespoons of *Benefiber* in 12oz glass of sugar-free ice tea	
1 cup *Egg Beaters* Garden Vegetable with 1 slice of *Nature's Own* whole wheat toast (which has 3 grams fiber /slice)	200
Mid-morning snack:	
One cup of raspberries	100
(raspberries are a high fiber fruit)	
Lunch:	
Lean Cuisine Swedish Meatballs	
Diet soft drink	
Sugar-free jell-o	290
Mid-afternoon snack:	
Low fat yogurt and fruit cup	90
Dinner:	
12" *Subway* Turkey sub with all veggies (no oil or cheese added. Mayo is ok since Subway uses fat free mayo)	600
Dessert:	
Dr. Phil's Shape Up Chocolate Peanut Butter Bar	210
Total Calories:	1490

All patients in my program whether on a qualitative or quantitative diet are on a multivitamin supplement and a dietary fiber supplement. For my patients, I recommend a multivitamin of their choosing and guar gum (*Benefiber*). Guar gum, in addition to its stool softening properties as a fiber supplement, also expands in your GI tract giving you a feeling of fullness longer thereby reducing your appetite (14). So why not use all the help you can get and "kick it up a notch" with the benefit guar gum provides to your weight loss effort.

Two things should be noted about guar gum though. The first is that guar gum won't help you lose weight unless its use is part of a greater weight management program (15). The second is that, in the past manufacturers of certain herbal weight loss medications utilized very high concentrations of guar gum in their supplements. This super-high concentration of guar gum led to a number of cases of gastrointestinal obstruction for people using them. The FDA has since banned its use in such high concentrations in weight loss pills. It is still routinely used as a food thickener, stool softener, and dietary fiber supplement. *Benefiber* is a great source of guar gum. It is virtually tasteless and odorless and is safe to use at the recommended dose labeled on the bottle. I recommend 2 tablespoons in water or beverage of your choice twice a day before breakfast and before dinner. My patients have often reported to me that this regimen helps reduce those mid-morning and late night cravings. Psyllium husk (Metamucil) is another source of natural dietary fiber that can be substituted for Benefiber for those who prefer. The dose is one tablespoon twice a day.

Let's talk a moment about calcium. I ensure all my weight loss patients have an adequate intake of calcium. The US recommended daily allowance for calcium is 1200 mg and for vitamin D (which is required for calcium absorption) is 400 IU. I generally recommend Oscal-D one tablet twice a day, which easily meets these requirements, or a nutritional equivalent. Recent studies have shown that obese patients on a high calcium diet lose up to 26% more weight than those whose diets are low in calcium (16). Calcium inhibits an enzyme called fatty acid synthase which resides in fat cells and helps promote synthesis of fat molecules, hence the name (17). This is the likely reason behind calcium's beneficial effects on our metabolism and why adequate intake is important for weight loss. In addition, calcium is also beneficial for osteoporosis prevention and may even protect against colon cancer. If you have certain medical conditions including kidney stones, renal failure, or parathyroid disease you'll need to consult with your doctor before starting calcium supplements.

Exercise is also an important part of weight management and good health in general. The American Heart Association recommends exercising at least four days a week for at least 30 minutes a day. This will not only help boost your metabolism but also improve your overall cardiovascular fitness, which basically means your heart will pump more efficiently even when not exercising. Even in people with normal weight, an overly sedentary, inactive lifestyle is an independent risk factor for heart disease. So you can tell your skinny friends that regular exercise will add years to their lives too. I recommend a good aerobic activity for my patients at least four times a week, an activity that gets their heart rate up and makes them sweat. That 'be accomplished through a brisk walk, a jog, 30 minutes on the exercise bike, a game of tennis, a swim, etc. Adding some resistance training (push-ups, sit-ups, arm curls, etc.) to your regimen for about 10 minutes twice a week will also be beneficial. Resistance training will add lean muscle mass to your body and help you burn more calories at rest since lean muscle requires more calories for daily maintenance than fat.

There are no more special details you need to know about exercise. You don't need to buy any fancy machines or weight loss gadgets, unless you want to. See what sport or exercise regimen fits best in your daily life and just implement that about four days a week. Some of my patients take their dog out for an extra 15 minutes during their walk to meet their exercise quota. Others have tennis buddies they meet on a regular basis. In addition, there are a number of very simple and easy behavioral modifications you can make to increase you body's energy expenditure through physical activity. We'll get to these in the chapter on behavioral principles.

That's all I'm going to say about diet selection and exercise. For the purposes of this book, there is no reason to go into too much detail about the various diets out there. Remember, diet selection is only one of the 6 steps, albeit an important one. You've probably heard about this topic a million times before. However, the important thing is that you now understand the key difference between a qualitative and quantitative diet, and you can use this understanding to categorize the various diets you've come across or tried in the past. You can use this information coupled with your own experience to help guide you through the process of diet selection. Think about the diets you have tried in the past. Were they quantitative or qualitative diets? Refer to table 7 for a quick category reference for some of the more popular diets out there.

Table 4 (Popular Diet Categories)

	Qualitative		Quantitative
	Low carb	Mod Carb	
The South Beach Diet*		X	
The Atkin's Diet	X		
The New Sugar Busters		X	
The Zone*		X	X
Protein Power	X		
The Fat Flush Plan*		X	X
USDA Food Pyramid			X
Weight Watcher's Diet			X
Dr. Phil's Ultimate Weight Solution			X

Author recommended diet is The South Beach Diet

The Zone Diet and The Fat Flush Plan are actually combined qualitative and quantitative diets

Choosing a diet is actually quite simple! From my point of view, if you don't have any of the previously mentioned chronic medical conditions, then I highly recommend purchasing **The South Beach Diet** and following it to the letter. It is very effective and loaded with food choices that are good for your health anyway. The pounds will melt away. If you are not a good candidate for the diet or a low-carb/modified-carb diet in general, then you'll need to break out your calculator because you have some calorie counting to do. You will need to utilize some form of portion controlled meal replacements (PCMR) to keep you honest. Remember, we generally underestimate our calories by 30% when we are on a quantitative diet. The Monarch Forever Fit program is a great comprehensive quantitative diet and fitness program which can be accessed online at http://www.monarchhealthsciences.com/2. Weight Watchers has a relatively good set up as well. Both can be quite costly overtime but may be well worth it. You can visit The American Heart Association's official website at: http://www.americanheart.org for further instruction on how to pursue a traditional balanced diet for weight loss. In general, most people will lose 1-2 pounds a week by consuming a 1500 calorie/day diet.

Now, let's move on to the next chapter and explore some of the cognitive barriers (mental misperceptions) to weight loss you never knew you had.

Part IV

Step 4: Cognitive Principles

Remember How I told you obesity is a multi-factorial disease. In this chapter, you're going to learn about how specific cognitive barriers have prevented you from losing weight in the past and keeping it off. We have thus far reviewed the importance of having a good medical exam and screening done by your doctor. This will ensure there are no medical barriers standing in the way of your weight loss and will also give you medical clearance to pursue active weight management. We have also gone over some important scientific concepts and physiology involved in weight management as well as diet selection and exercise.

A cognitive barrier can be defined as a mental misperception that acts to twist or misalign your understanding of something. The end result is essentially self-deception and misinterpretation of the facts. Psychologists often use cognitive therapy on their patients with clinical depression or clinical anxiety. Cognitive therapy basically involves retelling the story of a certain event to more represent the facts. We all have a tendency to overly generalize or delete positive aspects of certain bad experiences when we want to feel bad about ourselves for something.

An example might be a college student who performs poorly on an exam and later tells himself, "I'm stupid, I'll never do well in school." By saying this to himself a number of times he sets up a cognitive barrier for himself to prevent academic success. Subconsciously he has set up this new thinking to represent a false perception of reality. This is absolutely a wrong way to think, and if he does not crawl over the mental barrier he's created for himself his perceived reality may even come true! This is known as a "self-fulfilled prophesy."

The correct way to think about his recent poor test score would be the following:

1) I'm obviously smart enough to be in college so I'm not stupid.

2) Everyone fails a test now and then, even the best students.

3) What did I do wrong that I can correct in the future to prevent this from happening again?

The above statements represent the same story of the student's poor test performance but are actually much more accurate in representing the facts of what happened. By focusing on reality, this story eliminates emotional biases and prevents any cognitive barrier from forming.

The most important cognitive barrier you may have regarding weight loss is the thinking that, "I've failed so many times in the past, I'll never lose weight." This type of thinking is not only inaccurate but very destructive. You are responding emotionally to prior failure and are distorting reality. You have to stop thinking this way before you can move on with your weight loss. This is very important!

The reason you failed before is because you went about it wrong, not because you can't do it. This book will provide you with the correct methodology and this time you will succeed with both weight loss and weight maintenance. Remember, obesity is multifactorial, and you probably approached it only with diet and/or exercise alone in the past without regard to the other important steps involved.

Most patients who come to me for help with their weight have tried various diets in the past and have failed numerous times with either weight loss or maintenance of weight lost. They usually are very discouraged and are coming to me as a last ditch effort to accomplish what they perceive as "the impossible." So you can imagine that I spend a fair amount of time correcting their thinking with cognitive therapy.

I had a patient come to me with a BMI of 47 (severe obesity) who told me that she was doing everything right but not losing the weight. She was on a calorie counting diet (remember quantitative diet because you are counting something) and stated that she was only taking in 1500 calories/day and walking about 2 miles/day five days a week. I enrolled her in my program and did a thorough medical screening which showed there was nothing wrong with her body or metabolism that was preventing weight loss. So, I confronted her about this and discovered that the problem was not with her body, but with her mind. "There [was] no spoon" (*The Matrix*)

I explained to her that it was impossible for her not to lose weight if she was indeed only taking in 1500 calories and on top of that exercising regularly. I reviewed with her Einstein's Theory of

The Law of Conservation of Energy which tells us that energy cannot be created or destroyed. It only changes from one form to another. Calories act as little energy molecules in our body, and if we consume more than we use our body converts the extra calories into the form of fat cells for storage. So, either she was wrong in what she was telling me, or Einstein was wrong! When hearing the story told to her in this way she broke down in tears and then began admitting to me the things she had done wrong in the past. She also admitted that she was convinced it was impossible for her to ever lose weight. She actually believed this, as if something in the heavens predetermined she would always be heavy and there was nothing she could do about it! She is currently still enrolled in my program and is 40 pounds lighter. Her success underscores the importance of recognizing and eliminating cognitive barriers for a weight loss program to succeed.

Now that you know that weight loss is certainly in your grasp, particularly if you are using this book, let's talk about another disturbing, but common cognitive barrier. This one deals specifically with misperceptions of obesity as part of one's self-definition instead of as a disease that can be treated.

We generally use various characteristics to help our minds define and classify ourselves as well as other people. You may classify a person as tall or short; blond hair or dark hair; blue eyes or brown eyes; and fat or thin. It is this last classification as "fat or thin" where the problem lies. Your weight is in every respect a modifiable aspect of yourself and your being. All of the other classifications in the previous list are genetically determined, not permanently modifiable, and not considered disease states.

When you start looking at obesity for what it is, a disease, and not simply as a personal characteristic trait of your body, you open the door for change and improvement. You will realize that you need to play an active role in your own weight management. This is the case for most diseases out there.

For example, a diabetic patient is expected to play an active role in the management of his disease. This role often includes: taking medication, measuring blood sugars regularly, dietary modification, getting routine blood tests done, etc. The diabetic wouldn't accept his diabetes as just part of his body, like he would his height or his hair color for example, and do nothing about it (at least I hope he wouldn't)!

Obesity is a disease and it has reached epidemic proportions in our country. Obesity results in about 300,000 deaths per year in this country alone and the rates continue to rise. Take a look around you next time you are at the grocery store or shopping mall. Count the first twenty adults you see and calculate how many of those appear overweight or obese to you. I bet you'll get at least 50% almost every time.

The bottom line of this chapter is that: Obesity IS a disease and obesity CAN be treated. This is the new story to replace whatever story you had convinced yourself of in the past regarding your weight. We need to actively accept that obesity is a disease on both the individual and societal level and that this disease can be treated like many other common diseases out there. This book is your first step toward that end. Now that we got this all straightened out, let's move on!

Part IV

Step 5:
Behavioral Principles

In this chapter we're going to deal with another very important element of the weight management package known as behavioral modification. Behavioral modification is crucial to weight management but is often overlooked by your routine dieter (18,19). Your behavior is basically defined as your way of acting or reacting in your environment. Believe it or not, there are many environmental cues constantly acting around you causing you to behave in a repeated, conditioned way that is sabotaging your weight loss success. For the sake of brevity, I'm going to focus on the aspects of behavioral modification which I feel are the most practical and which have thus far worked very well for my patients losing weight. We're going to break this topic up into three subgroups:

1) Eating cues

2) Activity modification

3) Social support

Eating Cues

Conditional reflexes play an important role in determining our behavior. Our bodies and minds are constantly responding to various environmental cues that influence us in different ways. The 19th century Russian scientist Ivan Pavlov was the first to demonstrate the presence of environmental conditioning in his experiment on dogs.

Pavlov did an experiment involving dogs where he rang a bell every time he fed the dogs. After a while, the sound of the bell became the environmental cue for the dogs to eat, and they would salivate readying themselves for a meal every time they heard its sound. The bell cued them to eat even when food was not present.

Let's consider some examples of how our own environment affects us in particular ways. Certain color schemes may change your mood and make you feel a certain way. Soft, brightly mixed colors tend to be uplifting; whereas, dark, ashy colors can be depressing. Slow, rhythmic background music played in grocery stores cues you to slow down your pace spending more time in the store resulting in more shopping (grocery store owners know this)! In the case of ex-smokers, meeting old smoking buddies or visiting old smoking hangouts deliver many cues to smoke leading to overwhelming temptation to smoke again. On this same note, there exist many different environmental triggers that stimulate you to eat, even at times when you are not hungry.

These cues can be obvious things like feeling hungry after watching the cooking channel or having a "Big Mac Attack" after seeing a McDonald's commercial. You don't need my help identifying and dealing with these type of cues. I would like to focus on helping you find your own personal Pavlovian Bell, so to speak. That is to say, Pavlov was able to associate something completely unrelated to food like a bell tone to appetite stimulation. Each one of us has at least one or two crucial cues that act on us daily and cause us to desire food even when we're not hungry. These cues often have nothing to do with food itself and thus act as our own personal Pavlovian Bell driving us to eat. Once you discover your own Pavlovian Bell and modify your response to it accordingly you'll be amazed as to how much easier weight loss and weight maintenance will be. This is an important component of The 6-Step Methodology and should be taken seriously. Remember, obesity is multi-factorial, and we're going to attack it at every angle and therefore conquer it in the end!

In my experience with patients trying to lose weight, the most common Pavlovian Bells are the internal emotions of fatigue, boredom, depression, and stress. These emotional states are very powerful forces and can make or break your weight loss effort. All of us experience at least one of the above emotional states on a consistent basis in our daily lives, and they cause us to eat when we're not hungry. I think the reason is because high caloric, quick-fix food gives us a quick escape from the above negative feelings. Overtime our eating behavior has been adapted to accepting these states as eating cues, thus forming our own personal Pavlovian Bell.

My personal Pavlovian Bell is stress. I have two kids, a thriving medical practice, and an adventurous wife so I'm rarely bored. Fatigue and depression are also unusual for me. However, stress (both the good kind and the bad) is quite common and is a powerful force affecting my eating behavior. My first instinct when feeling stressed is to grab a quick-fix snack, which usually ends up being about 600 calories when I'm done. The way I've dealt with this is by keeping low calorie snacks around me during anticipated stressful situations, particularly long car trips with the kids. I now grab for diet soda and fat-free popcorn and end up eating 200 calories instead of 600.

There are a number of common external eating cues as well. These include sitting down in a movie theater, watching the big game on tv, or staying in on a rainy day. I think we're all familiar with the different type of cravings these situations bring about. Personally, my biggest external Pavlovian Bell is going to the movies. I immediately crave a big tub of popcorn with massive amounts of that liquid heaven you pour over it at the butter counter! It doesn't matter if I'm going to the movies right after dinner or on an empty stomach. It's always the same. Can you guess what I do to get around this situation? I'll leave that to your imagination. Let's just say my wife usually brings her big purse with her when we go to the movies.

What's your personal Pavlovian Bell? Try taking a few days and focus on the different environmental or emotional cues that bring you to eat even when you're not hungry. When you discover this about yourself you will have taken a big step toward weight loss. You can modify your response to these various cues to significantly reduce your calorie intake therefore taking control of your eating behavior. Maybe you'll snack on diet soda and fat-free popcorn like me. Maybe you'll chew gum instead or keep a tape player around and listen to your favorite song to make you forget about food. If you crave chips and a burger when you watch the game, try buying an assortment of raw veggies and keeping it out before the game begins. You'll naturally reach for it if it's right in front of you. As time goes on, you will have turned your modified response into a habit, and it will get easier and easier to avoid the unnecessary calorie intake when your Pavlovian bell calls to you.

Activity Modification

Now, let's talk a little bit about activity modification, the second important behavioral principle in weight management. As Americans, we live in one of the most modern, technologically advanced countries in the world. However, it's no coincidence that Americans are also among the most overweight people in the world. We live in a society of elevators, automobiles, remote controls, automatic doors, etc. These as well as other elements of the modern world can act as a trap for your weight loss effort by offering too much comfort and encouraging laziness (20). Consider the following examples.

How many of us have spent an extra 5 minutes in the car looking for the closest parking space at the grocery store or mall? By doing so we are wasting time, gas, and money as well as missing out on a very easy opportunity to burn calories (21). In most buildings elevators are so fast and comfortable that most people reflexively look to use them instead of the stairs.

My wife and I were in an airport one day going from the gate to the customs area which was about 300 meters away. We chose to walk instead of using the moving platform. Needless to say, we were one of the first people to arrive in customs having passed the 90% of people who chose the moving platform (most of whom were standing instead of walking). By over-relying on modern technology to do many of our day to day activities for us, we miss out on many opportunities to be more physically active and burn more calories.

Trying to maximize physical effort in your daily life is a practical and easy way to help boost your body's metabolism. Your body will burn calories during times you are used to being inactive. Think of this as the extra credit of weight loss. Remember, obesity is multi-factorial, and we need to hit it at every angle to have long term success. Let those people who really need the modern conveniences be the ones to use them. People with small children or who are medically injured should be the ones using elevators and parking close to buildings.

If you make it a habit to park further away, you'll not only do more walking in a day, but you'll probably get fewer dents in your car too. If you're ever at a grocery store and all the close spots are empty, you'll know that the other people in the store have read this book, and maybe you can strike up a conversation with them. You should also always use stairs whenever you are able to. Believe me, it's a great way to burn calories. One of my successful weight loss patients takes 15 minutes during his lunch break every day and walks up and down the stairs in his building. These are very easy modifications you can make in your daily activity that will go a long way for you in the long run, particularly with weight maintenance.

So, you now know to always park your car far away from your destination and to always use the stairs. What other activity modifications could you make in your day to day life to get more extra credit? Everyone has a different daily routine; so you'll have to think about this one and implement it on your own. It will be time well spent. Myself, I wrote 60% of this book standing using the kitchen counter instead of sitting at the table!

Social Support

Let's talk about the final topic under behavior modification, developing a social support system. Don't even think about trying to lose weight in secret! Many people hide the fact that they are dieting because of embarrassment about their weight. If you do this, it will definitely impair your chance for long term success. It is very important that those around you are aware of your weight loss effort so they can support you along the way. You'll be surprised how much your family and close friends will support you once they know you are on a concerted weight loss plan and know how important it is to you.

There will certainly be times where you experience temptation and perhaps even occasionally cheat on your diet. That is completely natural for anyone! However, you will need an external support system of people around you to reinforce your internal support during those times of difficulty. Reassurance from those around you will equip you to deal with temptation when it comes along. It will also help minimize your losses during times you gave in and cheated by helping you jump right back on the wagon! We are only human, and small failures here and there are part of our existence. It is how you recover from those tough times that will influence your weight loss success in the end.

Now, you may come across that occasional pushy relative or colleague who is always encouraging you to eat and to give up all that weight loss stuff! You just tell them that you are following your doctor's orders (coming straight from myself, Dr. Virji), and that you don't want to end up just another statistic. Obesity kills 300,000 people a year in this country and you are determined not to be one of those people. Obesity increases your risk for developing heart disease, stroke, cancer, stomach ulcers, and chronic infections to name a few. Remember, only you are the one (not that pushy relative or colleague of yours) who will face the consequences of letting your weight get out of control. So, just brush away those comments if you come across them and move on! Overall, you will find these types of people to be in the minority; most everyone else will support you.

You now know the major behavioral techniques which you need to lose weight and to keep it off. You need to find your eating cues and deal with them appropriately; modify your daily activities to work for you not against you; and develop a social support system for reinforcement. Pretty easy, right! Many studies out there show the positive effect of behavioral modification in long term weight loss; so take this part of your program seriously. Go ahead and start making these adjustments in your daily life; the only thing you have to lose is weight! Let's move on.

Part V

Step 6: Weight Maintenance

Congratulations! You've made it this far. You now know all you need to know to lose weight successfully. No fancy gadgets, fad diets, or hocus pocus necessary. You are now fully armed to battle your weight and win in the end. Obesity is a multi-factorial disease and needs to be addressed at all angles.

Step one: any medical barriers will be wiped away with your complete physical exam (CPE) and physician consultation. **Step two**: you understand the important neurologic hormones involved in controlling your weight and how to take control of them, as well as calculate your BMI and ideal body weight. **Step three**: You know how to choose a diet and develop an exercise program. **Step four**: You've broken down cognitive barriers that have sabotaged your weight loss in the past. **Step five**: you've modified your behavior to work for you not against you to achieve weight loss. Now it's time for **step six**, the most important of them all, weight maintenance. We're going to divide this step into four categories as follows:

1) Weight surveillance

2) Goal setting

3) Medical surveillance

4) Weight loss medication

Weight Surveillance

In order to maintain your weight successfully you need to be able to track your weight in an accurate way. Weighing yourself daily can sometimes be misleading. Weight may fluctuate throughout the day depending on such things as clothing, food intake, and time of the month for women.

A better way to go about weight surveillance is weighing yourself about three times a week. Then take the average weight and compare that number to the average of the week prior. This is a better, more accurate way to track your weight and also helps to avoid the common pitfall of "scale obsession." Many people weigh themselves on a daily basis, and the number that pops up on the scale basically determines their mood for the rest of the day. This number is not only very misleading but will lead you to a lot of anxiety since it will naturally fluctuate from hour to hour and day to day. You need to break out of this habit! Think of it this way, drinking a 16 oz bottle of water will cause that number to go up one pound. That extra weight is obviously not coming from your fat cells. When you relieve yourself 30 minutes later that weight will conveniently disappear.

Go out and buy a good scale. Weigh yourself in the morning about three times a week. Take the average number for the week and record it in a weight management journal so you can compare your weight from week to week to see how you are doing. Also, keep in mind that not all scales are the same. Weighing yourself at home and at the doctor's office may give you different numbers each time. That is not important. What is important is that your weekly averages are compatible with your weight management goals, whether you are in a maintenance cycle or losing cycle.

Goal Setting

Rome wasn't built in a day! You will not achieve your ideal body weight overnight. Your weight loss will be slow and gradual. Anyone who tells you otherwise is trying to sell you something. The good news is that if you stick to the principles in this book your weight loss will be permanent! Setting appropriate attainable goals is the first step to successful weight maintenance.

Let's go back to chapter two for a moment. Your body has this mechanism by which it tries to pull you back to a certain pre-set weight once you begin weight loss. It tries to accomplish this by means of a powerful neuro-hormone called leptin. Once your fat cells shrink and begin producing less leptin for your brain, your hypothalamus gets very irritated and works hard at stimulating your appetite trying to get you to return that stolen weight. You have to accept this as part of your body's natural physiology to preserve itself, and you have to work around it.

Studies have shown that with as little as a 10% loss of body weight you can achieve significant health benefits in multiple areas. This is a great starting point and will help us deal with leptin! Your weight management plan needs to be divided into two cycles: weight loss and weight maintenance. These are two very distinct things.

You will start with a weight loss cycle which begins after you put this book down. For your weight loss cycle you will work toward losing 10% of your body weight in about a three month period. For most people this will be between one and three pounds a week. You will successfully apply what you learned in steps one through five to achieve this goal. You will be attacking your obesity from every possible angle which will be a change from what you've done in the past, and you'll find that meeting this goal is easier than you think. It is important to follow each of the individual steps to the letter without cheating. Your initial goal weight will unlikely be your dream weight or ideal body weight. Remember, it's a marathon and this is just the first few laps.

After losing 10% of your body weight, your leptin receptors will be charged and ready to try and sabotage your weight loss effort. If you continue to run a full-court-press against your weight now, your leptin receptors will catch you in a crossfire leading back to the road to obesity (figure 6). At this point, you will need to end your first weight loss cycle and shift to your first weight maintenance cycle. Your weight maintenance cycle will also last three months.

It is very important to understand the difference between weight loss and weight maintenance. During weight maintenance your primary focus is on NOT gaining weight. This is very different than losing weight. By focusing on not gaining weight you are giving your body time to readjust to its new change. At the same time, you are readying yourself for the battle with leptin which happens to be at its height during the first 10% weight loss mark. You must realize that your goal is different in the weight maintenance cycle than in the weight loss cycle, and you must exercise patience if you want to achieve long term success.

Figure 6

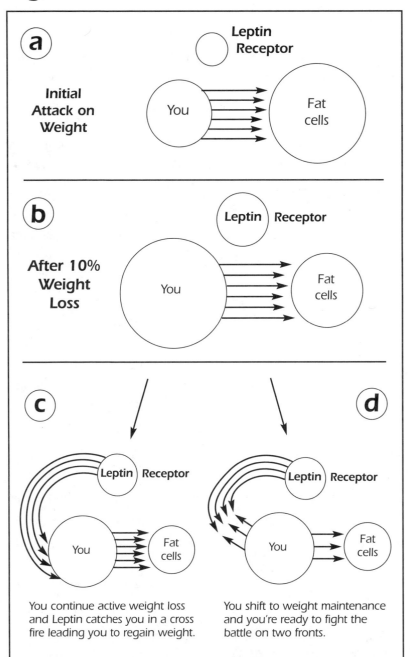

You continue active weight loss and Leptin catches you in a cross fire leading you to regain weight.

You shift to weight maintenance and you're ready to fight the battle on two fronts.

Weight maintenance is a lot less gratifying and socially rewarding than weight loss which is why it is so often neglected. During weight loss your clothes are starting to become loose, friends are noticing the difference and making comments toward you, and you generally feel great about yourself. These benefits are generally absent during weight maintenance leading you to forget about its importance. Do not fall into this trap! This is the time to stand your ground until reinforcements arrive. Focus on keeping your weight where it is for three months and avoid any guilt that you've stopped moving forward for a while. This is all part of the plan. During this time, your hypothalamus will eventually get the idea that this new weight is here to stay. It will downgrade its number of leptin receptors to accept this new lower concentration of leptin as its baseline and stop pushing you so hard to regain the weight (figure 7).* After this is achieved, no sooner than three months, you will be able to re-enter another weight loss cycle if desired.

Remember, all you need is a 10% loss of body weight to get a significant health benefit and add years to your life. When you've reached this point you have already achieved great success! However, if you wish to pursue further weight loss, then by all means, let's keep going and enter weight loss cycle number two. Just remember, you need every step in this book to make your changes permanent. Skipping steps will only harm you in the end. To enter weight loss cycle number two you'll need to start with step one again and take a trip to your doctor for another medical screening. Since we've already gone through one cycle we'll refer to this as medical surveillance.

---

* *The theory of hypothalamic receptor modulation over a period of time is generally the author's inference. The science of leptin physiology is relatively new and many studies continue in this area. It is well-accepted in the scientific community that slow-steady weight loss is safer and more sustainable than quick, immediate weight loss. In addition, receptor modulation in various organ systems secondary to various stimuli is a common physiologic phenomenon in the body. These are the basis of the author's inference regarding long-term hypothalamic receptor modulation.*

Figure 7

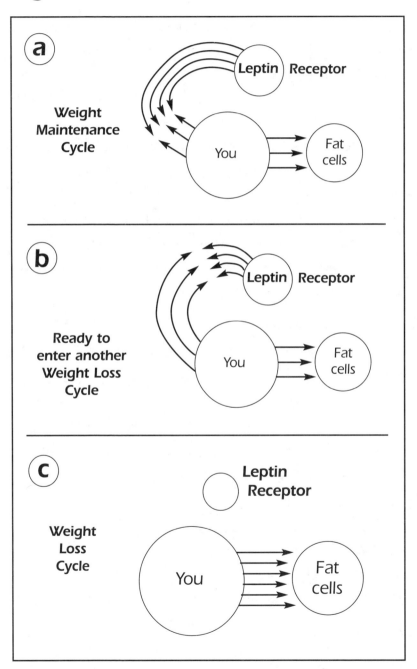

Medical Surveillance

Let's talk about medical surveillance. To do this we need to go back to step one for a moment. If you had any abnormal tests during your CPE including: high blood pressure, high bad cholesterol, low good cholesterol, elevated liver enzymes, or elevated glucose then the first thing you'll need once you've achieved 10% weight loss is to set up a follow-up appointment with your doctor (if all of these were normal and you have no other chronic medical problems you can skip this part). Ask him or her to retest any of the prior abnormal test results. You will see a significant change for the better! We know that obesity negatively affects just about every organ system in the body and with your initial weight loss you will see the difference for yourself. No need to take my word for it, seeing is believing!

If you are on a medication for blood pressure, diabetes, heart-burn, arthritis pain, or high cholesterol there is a possibility you can come off your medication or at least lower the dosage. After all, shedding pounds often helps you to shed medications too. You can only do this with the help of your doctor though and should never try to change your medications on your own.

Experiencing the improvement in any of the obesity related medical diseases will act as a very strong positive reinforcement tool. I've had to stop a number of medications on my weight loss patients, and they love it! This will help ensure your long term success and weight maintenance. By seeing the total benefit for your health overall, not just your self-esteem, it will be easier for you to combat future temptation toward overeating or inactivity. It will also ready you for another weight loss cycle if that is in your long term plan.

Weight Loss Medication

"To err is human." You are an individual doing your best to not only succeed at weight management, but also trying to succeed in life in general. However, sometimes life throws you a curve ball which has the potential to throw off your weight loss effort. This is where certain weight loss medications can be helpful, on the rare occasion that you need them. But medication can only be used as an adjunct to all the previous steps, not as a substitution.

If you notice yourself beginning to gain weight again, then its time to act! This is an emergency no different than a diabetic whose blood sugar starts crawling up. The long term consequences of both these diseases, obesity and diabetes, are the same. The first thing you must do is ask yourself why are you gaining weight? There are many things that could be potentially hindering you without you even considering their effect on your weight. Maybe you sprained your ankle and are unable to burn calories through exercise or activity modification. Maybe you've had a personal tragedy in the family which has been depressing you and slowing down your metabolism. Maybe you've been on the road and have found adherence to your diet particularly difficult. Or maybe the appetite cravings have just caught up with you, and you need a little help dealing with them.

Whatever the case, you must make every effort to ensure that the particular circumstance you're facing does not compromise your weight loss or weight maintenance. By actively and consistently applying the 6-Step Methodology, you should be able to recognize the barrier and quickly adjust to your new circumstance so it doesn't affect your weight. If all else fails, a short course of medication may give you the boost you need to get through a particularly tough time. You'll need your doctor's help with this.

There are two FDA approved medications to aid in long term weight loss, Sibutramine (*Meridia*) and Orlistat (*Xenical*). Sibutramine works as an appetite suppressant and also works to increase your metabolism. This can be used while on either a quantitative or qualitative diet. Orlistat works in your GI system by stopping your body's absorption of dietary fat and thus can only be used while on a low fat, quantitative diet. When used appropriately with the other steps in this book, these medications can help you sustain your weight loss in the long run.

In my clinic, I generally follow up with my patients every three weeks if in a weight loss cycle and every six weeks if in a weight maintenance cycle. If the weight starts creeping up, I do a thorough investigation to find out why and address the root cause first. This requires a return to the basics of the 6-Step Methodology and appropriate compensatory changes around the specific step where the deficiency lies.

Let's take some examples. Say you sprain your ankle and are unable to continue your walking regimen that you set up in Step 3 to meet your exercise requirement. In this case, you can modify your exercise regimen to include upper body resistance training (like push-ups and arm curls) instead of walking. You'll likely need to tighten up the diet a little to make up for the reduced calorie burning as well.   Let's take another example. Say you'll be on the road for a number of weeks making it difficult to stick to your diet. In that case, you can make sure you stay in a hotel that has a fitness facility and use that facility daily. You'll also be burning extra calories by using the stairs instead of the elevator to get to your room (but I didn't need to tell you that, right). If all else fails and you can't stop the weight gain, then maybe a short course of medication can help.

In a situation where despite my best efforts, the weight still continues creeping up, I'll begin my patient on a course of Sibutramine (*Meridia*) to help reestablish momentum and motivation during the difficult time for their weight management. Sibutramine has been shown in a number of studies to be a very useful and effective adjunct for weight loss (22, 23). I then titrate down the medication when they are ready to come off.

Weight management is a dynamic thing, and no two patients are the same. So my decision to use medication is highly individualized to the patient and circumstance of weight gain. Side effects of the medication must also be taken into consideration. If you have a history of heart disease or stroke then you won't be a candidate for Sibutramine. Orlistat will cause a lot of cramps, abdominal pain, and oily stools if you don't follow your low fat diet appropriately. Nevertheless, if you run into some difficulty with your weight loss or weight maintenance despite your best efforts, medications may help if you qualify to use them. You must be proactive and make an appointment with your doctor to help investigate why you're gaining weight and discuss the option of medication if needed. Don't wait to do this! A diabetic wouldn't wait until his blood sugar was in the lethal range before he sought help.

Let's talk a moment about over-the-counter weight loss remedies. As a general rule of thumb, you should avoid taking any over the counter diet pills! It does not matter whether they are advertised as nutritional supplements or otherwise. Most of them have not been tested for safety or efficacy and in reality there is no way of knowing what you are doing to your body. All over the counter preparations containing the once popular *Ephedra* (or ephedrine) diet supplement have been officially banned in the US as of April 12, 2004. Ephedra is a naturally occurring amphetamine- like compound extracted from the *Ephedra* species of plants including the ancient Chinese *Ma huang* and *Sida Cordifolia* to name a few. Ephedra supplementation has lead to the death of a number of athletes and results in an inappropriately high risk for stroke, heart attack, and sudden death syndrome.

Common commercial products like *Ripped Fuel Extreme* and *Triple Lean 3* contain a mixture of herbal preparations including Garcinia Cambogia, Coca seed extract, and caffeine. Few scientific studies are available to corroborate the hefty weight loss claim of many of these preparations. Some compounds including CLA (conjugated linoleic acid), carnitine, and green tea (catechins) have shown some modest weight loss benefit, but more studies are needed to confirm this effect as well as long-term safety.

There are even a number of natural preparations on the market that claim to help you lose weight by modulating your body's leptin or insinuating that they contain leptin. These preparations tend to be quite expensive as well. You should know that orally ingested leptin does not enter the brain so will have no influence on suppressing your appetite. Studies have failed to show a benefit of oral leptin supplementation on weight loss. Trust me, if it were that easy, I'd be the first one to tell you about it! So save your money. You're going to need it in about three months anyway, for your new wardrobe to replace all those large sizes that don't fit you anymore.

Part V

Conclusion

Congratulations! You've finished the book. You are now fully armed to combat your weight and never have it overtake you again. And you've learned all you need to know in record time. By utilizing the 6-Step Methodology you will be applying the best that both the old science and new science of weight management have to offer you. The choice to move on and take action is now yours. Don't hesitate and don't look back!

In the year 2000, $117 billion dollars was spent in this country treating obesity and obesity related diseases (24). That's money that could have been spent on tackling the unemployment issue, expanding health care to those without coverage, and feeding needy children. Speaking of children, the obesity crisis has not left them untouched. Fifteen percent of our nation's children and adolescents have reached the overweight mark, an all time high! Diseases like high blood pressure, high cholesterol, and diabetes which have traditionally been exclusive to the adult population have now hit our children at alarming levels (25). It was a very disturbing moment for me the first time I had to recommend a diabetic medication for an obese 10 year old.

Always remember that obesity is a disease, not a character trait. It has a multi-factorial etiology and needs to be addressed at every angle in order to be defeated. Each step in this book has a specific purpose, and each step must be understood and utilized thoroughly. If you didn't understand a certain section of the book, then go back and reread that section. There is no shame in that. Like my colleagues in medicine, I had to go through 11 years of training to become a physician. Believe me, during that time I had to reread many sections of many different books before I understood what was being taught.

It has been my privilege to assist you in your weight loss effort. As you can see, treating your weight not only has countless individual benefits, but benefits society as well. Be confident in that you now know all you need to know to lose weight and keep it off. Leave all excuses and cognitive barriers behind. You simply don't have time for those. Today is your day. Begin with changing your life, then go out and change the world! I wish you success and good health.

Part VI

Testimonials

Before I leave you, I thought it would be nice to give you some actual patient stories to demonstrate first-hand how The 6-Step Methodology works. These stories are based on patients who have been or who are currently enrolled in my weight management clinic. You'll see the importance of each individual step and how the six steps work synchronously over time to ensure successful weight management.*

Patient stories are based on actual patient cases. Names have been changed to protect patient confidentiality. Data for stories came from chart review and the author's memory. Direct patient consultation was made when it was available.

Tammy

Tammy is a great patient! She is very charismatic and is a successful entrepreneur. I first met her when she came to me for treatment of a respiratory infection. At that time, I noticed her blood pressure to be high which we followed-up on future visits. After a few more elevated readings it was clear that she needed to be on medication to control her blood pressure which had reached a whopping 160/112 (normal for most people is <140/90). It was time to confront her weight problem as well.

Her BMI was 47 (severely obese). When we discussed her weight, tears came to her eyes as she recounted stories of past failed weight loss attempts. She lost some weight on the Atkin's Diet in the past but gained it back. She also tried Weight Watchers without success as well as many other diets. She wanted a referral to a surgeon for bariatric surgery. Specifically, she wanted gastric bypass surgery (where they open up the abdomen and make major anatomical changes in the stomach and small intestine to promote weight loss). It was at that time I enrolled her in my weight management program. I convinced her to give The 6-Step Methodology a chance as a final effort to weight loss and weight maintenance. It was agreed that if I failed I would refer her to a bariatric surgeon.

We did a complete physical exam, medical screening, and appropriate lab work. She was determined not to be on blood pressure medication, and I informed her weight loss would be the key to that goal. She had no medical barriers in the way and was ready for aggressive weight management.

I taught her about BMI's, diet strategies, and leptin. She liked the idea of low glycemic index dieting and chose to be on The South Beach Diet. She continued her daily walking regimen and eventually hired a personal trainer to maximize her fitness goals. For her, initial cognitive restructuring was extremely important. Since she failed at weight loss so many times in the past, she had a cognitive barrier the size of The Berlin Wall and was certain that weight loss was not possible. But like The Berlin Wall, her cognitive barrier was dealt with and became a distant memory. Through cognitive restructuring she learned to treat obesity as a disease and not as a simple characteristic of her body. More importantly, she accepted that it was her responsibility to manage her weight the same way a diabetic needs to manage his blood sugar or a hypertensive needs to manage his blood pressure. Once we crossed the cognitive hurdle, the rest was downhill. Behavioral modification was quite easy as she had a naturally energetic and motivated personality.

She is currently 37 pounds lighter and feeling better than ever before. Her BMI has dropped from 47 to 40 and her current blood pressure is in the normal range at 130/80 without any medications. She bought a new sports car and is enjoying life with a renewed vigor. She is currently in a maintenance cycle and is soon to start losing more weight again.

Ronald

Ronald first came to me as a new patient for four different medical concerns, one of which was his weight. I dealt with the other three concerns, enrolled him in my program, and followed him over time for his obesity (original BMI 32). His job required him to be physically fit, and he was scared of being laid off from a lack of physical endurance which was secondary to his weight.

His medical screening demonstrated him to be hypothyroid, too little thyroid hormone circulating in his body. Low thyroid levels slow the body's metabolism and usually lead to weight gain. We fixed his thyroid level with medication, overcoming an important medical obstacle. Despite this, his weight still didn't budge. We reviewed important concepts of weight loss and selected a diet. He didn't like The South Beach Diet and preferred the Atkin's Diet which worked well for him in the past. He proceeded with a modified version of the Atkin's Diet which was lower in saturated fats; so I was ok with that.

Ronald was motivated from the start and knew he could lose weight. He didn't have any cognitive barriers and only needed a short review of behavioral modification techniques. In fact, he knew exactly what he needed. His particular problem was with snacking and cravings which he just couldn't control. They would come on progressively and consistently around the same time everyday. Ronald requested an appetite suppressant to help him with this particular dilemma. He was intelligent, had already begun his diet and exercise regimen, and was motivated to succeed. He just needed a little nudge. I prescribed him a course of Sibutramine to complement, not replace, his current weight loss effort. He is currently 17 pounds lighter and feeling great. He has job security, not to mention his blood pressure is down to 108/72 from 132/104 when we first met.

Les

Les struck me as a classic gentleman, timid yet very compassionate and quite intelligent. Nevertheless, he was also a classic "train wreck" patient the first time I met him. He had just about everything wrong with him including uncontrolled diabetes, high blood pressure, high cholesterol, liver disease (NASH), and venous stasis (chronic lower leg and feet swelling) to name a few. He was severely obese with a BMI of 44 which was contributing to most of his problems. He was treated by doctors in the past, but no one had aggressively pursued or emphasized the importance of long-term weight management with him.

He had a number of active medical issues we had to address during the process of weight loss. So his medical screening and medical surveillance took a lot more effort than most other people in my clinic. Nevertheless, this was contrasted with the fact that the other steps were relatively easy to apply with him. He picked up the medical concepts I taught him very quickly. He chose The South Beach Diet and adhered to it religiously, along with an active walking regimen. Despite his shy appearance, he really had only subtle cognitive barriers which were easily overcome. He developed a close support system of friends that encouraged him through his weight loss effort. Whenever he came for a clinic visit he always parked far away in the lot (next to me of course)!

He has lost a total of 32 pounds so far and is still going strong. His BMI is down from 44 to 39; so he has gone from the "severely obese" category to the "obese" category. Not only that, but his blood sugar and cholesterol are well-controlled. I had to cut his blood pressure pills in half because his weight loss had reduced his blood pressure down to 102/58. He didn't mind doing that at all!

References

1. Peeters A, Barendregt JJ, Willekens F, et al, for NEDCOM, the Netherlands Epidemiology and Demography Compression of Morbidity Research Group. Obesity in adulthood and its consequences for life expectancy: a life-table analysis. Ann Intern Med. 2003; 138: 24-32.

2. Calle, EE, Thun, MJ, Petrelli, JM, et al. Body-mass index and mortality in a prospective cohort of U.S. Adults. N Engl J Med 1999; 341:1097.

3. National Center for Health Statistics, Centers for Disease Control and Prevention, website www.cdc.gov/nchs/products/pubs/pubd/hestats/obese/obse99.htm (accessed April 20, 2004)

4. Friedman, XE, Reichmann, SK, Costanzo, PR, et al. Body image partially mediates the relationship between obesity and psychological distress. Obes Res 2002; 10:33-41.

5. Kennedy, A, Gettys, TW, Watson, P, et al. The metabolic significance of leptin in humans: gender-based differences in relationship to adiposity, insulin sensitivity, and energy expenditure. J Clin Endocrinol Metab 1997; 82:1293

6. Ostlund, RE Jr, Yang, JW, Klein, S, Gingerich, R. Relation between plasma leptin concentration and body fat, gender, diet, age, and metabolic covarities. J Clin Endocrinol Metab 1006; 81:3909.

7. NHLBI Obesity Education Initiative. Clinical guidelines on
    the identification, evaluation, and treatment of overweight
    and obesity in adults: the Evidence Report. NIH Publication
    No. 98-4083, U.S. Department of Health and Human Services,
    Public Health Service, National Institutes of Health, National
    Heart, Lung, and Blood Institute, Bethesda, MD 1998.

8. Choban, P, Atkinson, R, Moore, BJ. (Shape up America and the
    American Obesity Association.) Guidance for treatment of adult
    obesity, 1996: 1996-1998.

9. Samaha, FF, Iqbal N, Seshadri, P, et al. A low carbohydrate as
    compared with a low-fat diet in severe obesity. N Engl J Med.
    2003;348:2074-2081

10. Brehm BJ, Seely RJ, Daniels SR. A randomized trial comparing
    a very low carbohydrate diet and a low calorie-restricted low fat
    diet on body weight and cardiovascular risk factors in healthy
    women. J Clin Endocrinol

11. Lichtman, SW, Pisarska, K, Berman, ER, et al. Discrepancy
    between self-reported and actual caloric intake and exercize
    in obese subjects. N Eng J Med 1992; 327:1893

12. Wing RR, Jeffery RW. Food provision as a strategy to promote
    weight loss. Obes Res. 2001;9(suppl 4):271S-275S. Abstract

13. Flechtner-Mors, M, Ditschuneit, HH, Johnson, TD, et al.
    Metabolic and weight loss effects of long-term dietary interven-
    tion in obese patients: four-year results. Obes Res 2000; 8:399.

14. Kovacs, EM, Westerterp-Plantenga, MS, Saris, WH, et al. The effect of addition of modified guar gum to a low-energy semisolid meal on appetite and body weight loss. Int J Obes 2001;25:1. Abstract.

15. Pittlet, MH, Ernst, E. Guar gum for body weight reduction: meta-analysis of randomized tirals. Am J Med; 110:724-30[medline]

16. Zemel, Mb, Thompson, W, Milstead, A, et al. Calcium and dairy acceleration of weight loss and fat loss during energy restriction in obese adults. Obes Res. 2004; 12:582-590.

17. Zemel M. Role of Calcium and dairy products in energy partitioning and weight management. Am J Clin Nut 79; 5:907S-912S.

18. Foreyt, JP, Goodrick, GK. Evidence for success of behavior modification in weight loss and control. Ann Intern Med 1993; 119:698. Abstract

19. Hu, FB, Li, YL, Colditz, GA, et al. Television watching and other sedentary behaviors in relation to risk of obesity and type 2 diabetes melitis in women. JAMA 2003; 289:1785-1791

20. Levine, JA, Schleusner, SJ, Jensen, MD. Energy Expenditure of nonexercise activity. Am J Clin Nutr 2000; 72:1451.

21. Anderson, RE, Wadden, TA, Bartlett, SJ, et al. Effects of lifestyle activity vs structured aerobic exercise in obese women. JAMA 1999; 281:335.

22. Wadden TA, Berkowits RI, Sarwer DB, Prus-Wisniewski R, Steinberg C. Benefits of lifestyle modification in the pharmacologic treatment of obesity: a randomized trial. Arch Intern Med. 2001;161:218-227.

23. Arterburn, DE, Crane, PK, Veenstra, DL, et al. The efficacy and safety of Sibutramine for weight loss. Arch Intern Med. 2004; 164:994-1003.

24. Wolf AM, Colditz GA. Current estimates of the economic cost of obesity in the United States. Obes Res 1998;6:97-106.

25. Must A, Anderson SE. Effects of obesity on morbidity in children and adolescents. Nutr Clin Care 2003;6:4-12.

Verona Publishing, Inc.
P.O. Box 24071
Edina, Minnesota 55424

www.veronapublishing.com